FACING BREAST CANCER

Understanding Risks, Effects and Prevention

By Kayla Russell

DISCLAIMER

Copyright © by Kayla Russell 2024. All rights reserved.

TABLE OF CONTENTS

CHAPTER 1: *What is Breast Cancer?*

Introduction to Breast Cancer

Breast cancer remains a significant global health challenge, affecting millions of individuals and families each year. While considerable progress has been made in the understanding and treatment of breast cancer, new challenges, and trends continue to emerge, shaping the landscape of breast cancer care and research.

In recent years, advancements in technology and medical research have led to more personalized approaches to breast cancer treatment, allowing for tailored therapies based on individual characteristics and genetic profiles. Additionally, increased awareness and advocacy efforts have resulted in improved screening rates and early detection, leading to better outcomes for many individuals diagnosed with breast cancer.

However, despite these advancements, disparities in breast cancer outcomes persist, with certain populations facing greater barriers to access to care and resources. Socioeconomic factors, race, ethnicity, and geographic location can all impact breast cancer outcomes, highlighting the need for targeted interventions and equitable access to quality care.

Furthermore, emerging trends such as the rise of triple-negative breast cancer and the increasing prevalence of young women diagnosed with breast cancer underscore the evolving nature of the disease and the importance of ongoing research and innovation in the field.

In this chapter, we will explore the fundamentals of breast cancer, examine current trends and challenges, and discuss the impact of these developments on individuals and communities. By staying informed about the latest trends and advancements in breast cancer care, we can empower readers to make informed decisions about their health and well-being.

Join us as we embark on a journey to demystify breast cancer, raise awareness, and support those affected by this disease. Together, we can work towards a future where breast cancer is not only treatable but preventable, ensuring better health and well-being for generations to come.

What is Cancer

An illness known as cancer occurs when somebody's cells proliferate out of control and invade other bodily regions.

With trillions of cells making up the human body, cancer can begin practically anywhere. Human cells typically divide to create new cells as needed by the body by growing and multiplying. New cells replace old ones when they die as a result of aging or injury.

This controlled mechanism can occasionally malfunction, causing damaged or aberrant cells to proliferate and expand when they shouldn't. Tumors are lumps of tissue that can be formed by these cells. Cancerous or benign tumors can both occur.

Malignant tumors can metastasize, or spread into, neighboring tissues, and can also generate new tumors by traveling to far-off regions of the body. Malignant tumors are another term for cancerous tumors. Blood malignancies, including leukemias, typically do not develop into solid tumors, although many cancers do.

Benign tumors do not penetrate or spread to neighboring tissues. Benign tumors seldom grow back after removal, while malignant tumors occasionally do. However, benign tumors can occasionally grow to be rather enormous. Some, like benign brain tumors, are potentially fatal or cause severe symptoms.

What is Breast Cancer

The three basic components of a breast are connective tissue, ducts, and lobules. The glands that generate milk are called lobules. The tubes that transport milk to the nipple are called ducts. Everything is encased in and held together by the fibrous and fatty connective tissue.

Breast cancer is a condition when the breast's cells proliferate uncontrollably. Breast cancer comes in various forms. Which breast cells develop into cancer determines the type of breast cancer.

Most cases of breast cancer start in the lobules or ducts. Blood and lymph vessels are two ways that breast cancer can travel outside of the breast. Breast cancer is considered to have metastasized when it extends to other bodily parts.

The illness known as breast cancer is caused by aberrant breast cells that proliferate and develop into tumors. Tumors have the potential to grow throughout the body and become lethal if ignored.

Signs and Symptoms of Breast Cancer

Different people experience breast cancer in different ways. Some persons exhibit neither symptoms nor signs at all.

Among the early signs of breast cancer are:

- A newly discovered lump in the armpit or breast.

- Partially swollen or thickened breast tissue.

- Skin irritation or dimpling around the breasts.

- Flaky or red skin around the breasts or nipples.

- Pulling inward or experiencing pain in the nipple region.

- Blood or other types of breast milk-like discharge.

- Any modification to the breasts' size or form.

- Any kind of pain in the breast.

Remember that these symptoms are not exclusive to cancer. They can also occur with other illnesses.

See your doctor as soon as possible if you experience any symptoms or indicators.

What Is a Normal Breast?

A breast is not normal. For another woman, what is typical may not be normal for you. The majority of women report feeling uneven or lumpy breasts. Having children, losing or gaining weight, receiving your period, and taking certain medications can all have an impact on how your breasts feel and look. As you age, your breasts also tend to change.

What Do Lumps in My Breast Mean?

Breast lumps can be caused by a variety of illnesses, including cancer. However, the majority of breast lumps are brought on by other illnesses. Cysts and fibrocystic breast disease are two prevalent causes of breast lumps. Breast lumps, tenderness, and soreness can be caused by noncancerous changes brought on by fibrocystic disease. Cysts are tiny sacs filled with fluid that can form in the breast.

SUMMING UP

Breast cancer is a global health challenge that affects millions of individuals and families annually. Advancements in technology and medical research have led to personalized treatments, improved screening rates, and early detection, but disparities persist due to socioeconomic factors, race, ethnicity, and geographic location.

Breast cancer occurs when cells proliferate uncontrollably and invade other bodily regions. It can begin anywhere and can be caused by aberrant breast cells that proliferate and develop into tumors. Malignant tumors can metastasize or spread to neighboring tissues, while benign tumors do not penetrate or spread to neighboring tissues.

Symptoms of breast cancer include a newly discovered lump in the armpit or breast, partially swollen or thickened breast tissue, skin irritation or dimpling around the breasts, flaky or red skin around the breasts or nipples, pulling inward or experiencing pain in the nipple region, blood or other types of breast milk-like discharge, any modification to the breasts' size or form, and any kind of pain in the breast.

A normal breast is uneven or lumpy, and it can be affected by various factors such as having children, losing or gaining weight, receiving your period, and taking certain medications. Breast lumps can be caused by a variety of illnesses, including cancer, but are more common in women with cysts and fibrocystic breast disease. By staying informed about the latest trends and advancements in breast cancer care, readers can empower themselves to make informed decisions about their health and well-being.

CHAPTER 2: *Breast Cancer Causes and Risks*

What are Breast Cancer Risk Factors and Causes?

When certain processes that regulate cell development and division are rendered inoperable by mutations or changes in the DNA of breast cells, breast cancer results. These mutant cells frequently perish or come under attack by the immune system. Yet, some cells manage to elude the immune system, proliferate unchecked, and eventually develop into breast tumors.

The secret to reducing your risk of breast cancer is to prioritize the controllable risk factors and take proactive measures to monitor the unavoidable risk factors.

Numerous factors contribute to your risk of breast cancer, according to studies. The two biggest factors affecting your risk are becoming older and being a woman. Women 50 years of age or older are the ones who get breast cancer most often.

Some women will get breast cancer even in the absence of any other known risk factors. You do not automatically get the disease just because you have a risk factor, and not all risk factors have the same impact. Although the majority of women have some risk factors, most do not develop breast cancer. Discuss risk reduction strategies and breast cancer screening with your physician.

How Common is Breast Cancer?

According to the American Cancer Society (ACS), a woman's lifetime risk of acquiring breast cancer is approximately 13 percent. This corresponds to a 1 in 8 risk of breast cancer. It also indicates that you have a 7 in 8 chance of not getting breast cancer.

One in three cancers affecting women is breast cancer. According to the American Cancer Society, there has been a 0.5% annual increase in the risk of breast cancer in women in recent years.

What are the Risk Factors for Breast Cancer?

Risk factors are traits and circumstances that raise your chance of contracting an illness. Certain risk factors for breast cancer, such as being a woman, growing older, and having a family history of the disease, are unavoidable. To help reduce your chance of getting breast cancer, you can alter a few other risk factors. Physicians are baffled as to why some women with risk factors never develop breast cancer, while other women who have no risk factors other than being female do. However, you can try to reduce your risk by adopting specific lifestyle choices.

Risk Factors (Life Behaviors) that you can Manage

Drinking Alcohol

Every drink you take increases your risk of breast cancer. According to research, women who consume one alcoholic drink per day are seven to ten percent more likely to develop breast cancer than nondrinkers; for those who have two or three alcoholic drinks per day, the risk increases to twenty percent.

Lower your risk: One drink per day is considered moderate drinking for women. If you drink every day, start by reducing your consumption to a few occasions each week. Additionally, start tracking your alcohol intake. A typical drink contains roughly 14 grams of alcohol, or 12 ounces of ordinary beer, 5 ounces of wine, or 1.5 ounces of distilled spirits. One drink may count as two if it's filled into an enormous glass.

Your Weight

Among the illnesses and ailments brought on by or made worse by being overweight or obese after menopause is breast cancer. After menopause, your ovaries stop producing estrogen, the female sex hormone, thus adipose tissue is where most estrogen is found. Your body produces more estrogen the more fat you have, and estrogen feeds some breast tumors, enabling them to spread. Diabetes and breast cancer have been related to elevated blood insulin levels, which overweight women may also have.

Lower your risk by consulting a dietician to create a fruit- and vegetable-rich weight-loss plan that fits your schedule and increases the likelihood that you'll follow it through. Maintaining a healthy weight is very beneficial. After 50, women who maintain their weight loss are less likely to develop breast cancer than those who gain it again. Additionally, your risk decreases as you lose more weight. A large study published in the Journal of the National Cancer Institute found that women who lost between 4.4 and 10 pounds had a 13 percent lower risk of breast cancer than women who didn't lose weight, 16 percent lower risk for those who lost between 10 and 20 pounds, and 26 percent lower risk for those who lost more than 20 pounds.

A Sedentary Lifestyle

Your Risk of Breast Cancer Increases with Decreased Mobility.

Lower the risk: Maintaining an active lifestyle may help lower your risk of breast cancer and other diseases, as well as support your efforts to lose weight. According to the American Cancer Society, you should try to get 150–300 minutes per week of moderate-intense exercise, like brisk walking, or 75–150 minutes of more strenuous exercise, like jogging. The benefits increase with the amount of physical exercise you engage in. Consult your physician before making any significant adjustments to your fitness routine.

Risk Factors to take into Account

Your Past Reproductive Experiences

Women who are childless or whose first child was born after the age of thirty may be at a slightly increased risk of breast cancer. This is because longer lengths of time expose breast tissue to higher levels of estrogen. Women who become pregnant at an earlier age and have more births have a lower chance of developing breast cancer.

What to do: When thinking about your screening and preventive plan for breast cancer, talk to your doctor about your reproductive history.

Late Menopause/Early Menstruation

Because your breast tissue has been exposed to estrogen for a longer period, if you began menstruation before the age of twelve, you have an increased risk of developing breast cancer. For identical reasons, entering menopause later in life (beyond age 55) also increases the risk.

What to do: When discussing your options for breast cancer screening, bring up your menstrual history with your doctor.

No Prior Experience Nursing

Breastfeeding may lower your chance of breast cancer, particularly if you do it for a year or more. Breastfeeding offers numerous advantages, one of which is the prevention of breast cancer. According to the American Academy of Pediatrics, breastfeeding should be continued for at least a year after the first six months of life, with appropriate meals added as needed.

What to do: If at all possible, try breastfeeding your child as it also shields them from a variety of illnesses.

Hormone Consumption

Hormones are used in several birth control methods, which increases the risk of breast cancer. These could consist of:

- Oral contraceptives

- injection of birth control

- implants for birth control

- IUDs, or intrauterine devices

- Skin patches for birth control

- Rings in the vagina

Breast cancer risk increases with combination hormone therapy used after menopause. The possibility that the cancer will be discovered at a more advanced stage is also increased by combined HT.

What to do: Talk to your doctor about your worries and consider all the advantages and disadvantages before choosing hormone replacement medication or birth control.

Potential Risk Factors

Be mindful of unknown risk factors for breast cancer, such as high-fat diets, specific pesticides, and chemicals in personal care items. Additionally, some data suggest a higher risk of breast cancer is associated with night shift work. These possible risk factors are being intensively researched by researchers.

Other factors, such as wearing underwire bras, using antiperspirants, and having an abortion, have been substantially disproven by science. A common concern among women is the possibility of breast cancer and hair dye. The National Cancer Institute claims that despite a study of data from 14 studies, there is insufficient evidence to conclude that women who use hair color are more likely to develop breast cancer than those who do not.

Talk to your doctor about your risk factors at your next appointment to be sure you're taking all the precautions possible to avoid breast cancer. During your appointment, you may study one of the assessment tools to determine how likely you are to get breast cancer over the following five years and in your lifetime.

Your doctor may recommend early screening, more frequent or extensive screening, and possibly treatment if you are at an elevated risk.

Risk Factors Beyond Your Control

Which Gender Are You?

Although it's unusual, men can get breast cancer. Women are far more vulnerable.

What to do: Pay attention to the risk factors that you can alter, such as eating a healthy weight and exercising frequently.

Your Age

The risk of breast cancer increases with age. Women over 55 are the ones who typically develop breast cancer.

What to do: While routine mammography screening tests for breast cancer won't prevent the disease, they may detect it early on, when it's more treatable. Talk to your doctor about the ideal time for your breast cancer screening.

Your Family History

It is not a family history that predisposes you to breast cancer. Only 15% of patients report having a family relative with this illness. Having said that, you are deemed to be at an increased risk if you have first-degree relatives—parents, siblings, or children—who have a history of cancer.

What to do: Your risk is nearly doubled if your mother, sister, or daughter has breast cancer. If two of your first-degree relatives have breast cancer, your risk rises by around three times. Your risk is also increased if your father or sibling has breast cancer. The Centers for Disease Control and Prevention (CDC) claim that having a first- or second-degree relative with high-grade prostate cancer also puts you at a slightly increased risk.

Make sure your decisions for breast cancer screening take your family history into account.

Seeing a genetic counselor and getting tested for known breast cancer genes might be a good idea.

Your Genetic Makeup

Gene alterations or mutations inherited from your parents, such as the BRCA1 and BRCA2 mutations, may account for up to 10% of breast cancers. Scientists are searching for more genes that could contribute to the risk of breast cancer.

What to do: Consult a genetic counselor regarding the possibility of testing for the identified genes linked to breast cancer. For people of Ashkenazi Jewish origin, genetic counseling and/or testing for BRCA gene mutations are recommended. Talk to your doctor about medication or surgery alternatives if you have these mutations to lower your risk. For instance, the American Cancer Society states that a prophylactic bilateral mastectomy can lower your risk of breast cancer by 90 percent or more.

Your Individual Breast Cancer History

You have an increased risk of developing a new cancer in the other breast or a different area of the same breast if you have previously been diagnosed with breast cancer. This is seen as fresh breast cancer rather than a recurrence.

What to do: To keep an eye on this risk, adhere to the monitoring guidelines provided by your oncology team. Consult your physician about seeing a genetic counselor.

Your Race and Ethnicity

The highest lifetime risk of breast cancer is seen in White and Black women. The incidence of breast cancer in Asian/Pacific Islander and Hispanic/Latina women lies in the middle of the two main categories, but American Indian and Alaska Native women had the lowest risk.

White women are often more likely than Black women to get breast cancer, but they typically receive a diagnosis later in life (between 60 and 84). Among women under 40, black women had the highest incidence of breast cancer. A greater proportion of triple-negative breast cancer cases are found in black women.

What to do: To increase your chances of detecting cancer early, if your race or ethnicity puts you at increased risk, be sure to heed all screening guidelines.

Your Height

Compared to their shorter counterparts, taller women have a higher chance of developing breast cancer. Scientists are unsure of the cause of this phenomenon.

The Density of your Breasts

Dense breasts are believed to have a higher risk of developing breast cancer because they include more glandular and fibrous tissue and less fatty tissue. Additionally, breast tumors may be more difficult to see on mammograms in cases of dense breast tissue.

What to do: Consult your doctor about the best screening methods if you have dense breasts, as this needs to be documented in your medical records. This could involve not just mammograms but also other imaging modalities.

Benign Breast Diseases

Breast cancer risk may be increased by some non-cancerous breast diseases. Proliferative lesions without aberrant cell growth, such as fibroadenomas, sclerosing adenosis, multiple papillomas, and radial scars, are included in the list. Atypical ductal hyperplasia and atypical lobular hyperplasia are two examples of proliferative lesions with cell abnormalities that raise the risk.

How to proceed: Information is power. Make sure your doctor is aware of any past benign breast issues you may have had, and that information is taken into account when determining the best time and method for you to have a breast cancer screening.

Radiation to Your Chest

You might be more susceptible to breast cancer if you underwent radiation therapy to the chest as part of your treatment for another type of cancer.

What to do: When creating a screening strategy for breast cancer, take into account any history of radiation to the chest.

The Amount of DES you are Exposed to

A medication called DES, which mimics estrogen, was administered to some pregnant women in an attempt to reduce the risk of miscarriage between the 1940s and the early 1970s. Breast cancer risk may be elevated in mothers who use it, and maybe in their offspring as well.

What to do: Let your doctor know if you or your mother took DES to prevent miscarriage and talk about how it affects your screening schedule.

What is Considered a High Risk for Breast Cancer?

The following conditions, according to the CDC, increase your risk of developing breast cancer:

strong maternal, sibling, or child history of breast cancer in the family. Cancer risk is higher in both genders when there is a family history.

Hereditary modifications to your BRCA1 and BRCA2 genes

You run a high risk of developing ovarian cancer as a result of these two risk factors. Consult your physician about ways to lower your risks. Preventive surgery and medications that reduce or inhibit estrogen in the body are options.

When Cancer Spreads

Metastatic cancer is a type of cancer that has spread to various parts of the body from its original site. Metastasis is the process by which cancer cells move to different areas of the body.

The initial, or primary, cancer and metastatic cancer share the same name and type of cancer cells. For instance, breast cancer that spreads to the lung and develops into a tumor is called metastatic breast cancer, not lung cancer.

Metastatic cancer cells often have the same appearance as the initial cancer cells under a microscope. Furthermore, certain molecular characteristics, such as the presence of particular chromosome alterations, are typically shared by the original cancer cell and metastatic cancer cells.

Treatment may, in certain circumstances, help patients with metastatic cancer live longer. In other instances, stopping the cancer's spread or reducing its symptoms are the main objectives of treatment for metastatic cancer. The majority of cancer deaths are due to metastatic disease, and metastatic tumors can seriously impair a person's ability to operate.

SUMMING UP

Breast cancer is a disease caused by mutations or changes in the DNA of breast cells, which can either perish or be attacked by the immune system. The two biggest risk factors are becoming older and being a woman, with women aged 50 years or older being the most common carriers.

Risk factors for breast cancer include being a woman, growing older, and having a family history of the disease. To reduce your risk, you can adopt specific lifestyle choices. Drinking alcohol increases your risk of breast cancer, with women who consume one drink per day being seven to ten percent more likely to develop it than nondrinkers.

Being overweight or obese after menopause can also increase your risk of breast cancer. Consult a dietician to create a fruit- and vegetable-rich weight-loss plan that fits your schedule and increases the likelihood of following it through. Maintaining a healthy weight is beneficial, as studies have shown that women who lose between 4.4 and 10 pounds have a 13 percent lower risk of breast cancer than those who gained it again.

A sedentary lifestyle may help lower your risk of breast cancer and other diseases, as well as support your efforts to lose weight. Engaging in 150-300 minutes of moderate-intensity exercise per week can help lower your risk.

For women who are childless or have had multiple pregnancies, their reproductive history may be at a slightly increased risk of breast cancer due to longer exposure to higher levels of estrogen. When considering screening and preventive plans for breast cancer, talk to your doctor about your reproductive history.

Breast cancer risk is influenced by several factors, including late menopause, early menstruation, breastfeeding, hormone consumption, potential risk factors, and genetic makeup. Early menstruation and entering menopause later in life increase the risk of developing breast cancer. Breastfeeding may lower the risk, especially if continued for at least a year after the first six months of life. Hormone consumption in birth control methods, such as oral contraceptives, injectables, IUDs, skin patches, and rings in the vagina, also increases the risk. Combination hormone therapy used after menopause also increases the risk of breast cancer.

Potential risk factors include high-fat diets, pesticides, and chemicals in personal care items. Night shift work and wearing underwire bras have been disproven by science. Hair dye is a common concern among women, but there is insufficient evidence to conclude that women using hair color are more likely to develop breast cancer.

Risk factors beyond control include gender, age, family history, and genetic makeup. Women over 55 are more vulnerable to breast cancer, and routine mammography screening tests can detect the disease early. Genetic counseling and testing for known breast cancer genes may also be beneficial. Genetic counseling and/or testing for BRCA gene mutations are recommended for Ashkenazi Jewish individuals.

Breast cancer risk can be influenced by various factors, including individual history, race and ethnicity, height, breast density, benign breast diseases, radiation therapy to the chest, and exposure to DES. Individuals with a history of breast cancer or hereditary modifications to the BRCA1 and BRCA2 genes are at a higher risk of developing breast cancer.

Their breasts may have dense breasts, which may make it difficult to see on mammograms. It is important to consult a doctor about the best screening methods for dense breasts and to consider any history of radiation therapy. Additionally, DES, a medication that mimics estrogen, may be used to prevent miscarriage in some pregnant women.

High-risk individuals may also have a strong maternal, sibling, or child history of breast cancer in the family and have hereditary modifications to their BRCA1 and BRCA2 genes. Preventive surgery and medications that reduce or inhibit estrogen in the body can help lower these risks.

Metastatic cancer, which has spread to various parts of the body from its original site, can be treated in some cases to help patients live longer or to stop the cancer's spread or reduce symptoms. The majority of cancer deaths are due to metastatic disease, and metastatic tumors can significantly impair a person's ability to operate.

CHAPTER 3: *Test and Diagnosis*

Diagnosis of Breast Cancer

Exams and conversations about symptoms are frequently the first steps in the diagnosis of breast cancer. Imaging studies can examine breast tissue to look for abnormalities. A sample of breast tissue is taken for testing to determine whether or not cancer is present.

Breast Examination

A medical specialist examines the breasts during a clinical breast exam to check for anything unusual. This could involve modifications to the nipple or skin. The medical practitioner then palpates the breasts to check for lumps. The medical practitioner also palpates the area under the arms and along the collarbones for bumps.

Mammogram

An X-ray of the breast tissue is called a mammography. Mammograms are frequently used as a breast cancer screening tool. You may be scheduled for follow-up mammography to examine the area in further detail if the results of your screening mammogram are alarming. A diagnostic mammogram is a more thorough kind of mammography. It's frequently used to examine both breasts up close.

Breast Ultrasound

Sound waves are used in ultrasound technology to create images of internal body components. Your medical team may be able to learn more about a breast lump from a breast ultrasound. An ultrasound, for instance, could reveal whether the bump is a cyst filled with fluid or a solid tumor. Using this information, the medical team determines what more tests you might require.

MRI of the Breast

Radio waves and a magnetic field are used by MRI equipment to produce images of the inside of the body. More detailed images of the breast can be obtained with a breast MRI. This technique is occasionally performed to thoroughly inspect the affected breast for any additional cancerous growth. It may also be utilized to check for breast cancer in the other breast. You normally receive an injection of dye prior to your breast MRI. The tissue appears more prominent in the photos thanks to the dye.

Taking a Sample of Breast Cells for Testing

The process of taking a tissue sample for laboratory analysis is called a biopsy. A medical practitioner inserts a needle through the skin and into the breast tissue to obtain a sample. The medical practitioner uses ultrasound, X-ray, or other imaging technology to create images that are used to guide the needle. The medical expert uses the needle to remove tissue from the breast once it has reached the proper location. The location where the tissue sample was taken out is frequently marked with a marking. Tests using imaging technology will reveal the little metal tracer. The marker aids in the region of concern's monitoring by your healthcare team.

Testing Cells in the Lab

A biopsy tissue sample is sent to a lab for analysis. Tests can determine whether the sample's cells are malignant. Additional tests provide details about the kind of cancer and its rate of growth. Additional information about the cancer cells is provided by special testing. For instance, examinations may search for hormone receptors on the cell surface. The outcomes of these tests are used by your healthcare team to formulate a treatment plan.

Breast Cancer Types

Breast cancer comes in a wide variety of forms, which are determined by the site of the tumor's initiation in the breast, its growth or spread, and specific characteristics that affect the tumor's behavior. Together with your physician, you may select the most appropriate course of therapy for your particular kind of breast cancer by understanding the diagnosis.

Learn about the various forms of breast cancer, its molecular subgroups, breast cancer in men, and malignant phyllodes tumors of the breast here.

Breast Cancer: Invasive Versus Non-Invasive

The lobules, or milk-producing glands, or the ducts, or the passageways that carry milk from the lobules to the nipple, are typically where breast cancer starts. Details regarding the malignancy, such as whether it has progressed beyond the original breast lobules or milk ducts, are included in your pathology report.

Invasive Breast Cancer

Breast cancer that has spread into the surrounding breast tissue is referred to as invasive (or infiltrating). The two most prevalent forms of invasive breast cancer are distinguished by the location of their initiation in the breast:

IDC, or Invasive Ductal Carcinoma

The most prevalent kind of breast cancer is invasive ductal carcinoma (IDC), also known as infiltrating ductal carcinoma. Roughly 75% of all cases of breast cancer are IDCs.

When a cancer is invasive, it affects the breast tissues around it. Ductal refers to the cancer that originated in the tubes that bring milk from the lobules to the nipple, known as the milk ducts. Any cancer that starts in the skin or other tissues covering internal organs, like breast tissue, is referred to as a carcinoma. According to the American Cancer Society, there will be roughly 287,850 new instances of invasive breast cancer identified in women in 2022, with IDC accounting for the majority of these occurrences.

ILC, or Invasive Lobular Carcinoma

The type of invasive breast cancer known as invasive lobular carcinoma (ILC) originates in the lobules, which are the milk-producing glands in the breast. Invasive lobular carcinomas account for around 10% of all invasive breast cancer cases, making it the second most frequent kind of the disease.

Breast cancer that originates in the lobules—the milk-producing glands in the breast—is known as invasive lobular carcinoma (ILC). When a cancer is invasive, it affects the breast tissues around it. Any cancer that starts in the skin or other tissues covering internal organs, like breast tissue, is referred to as a carcinoma.

DCIS, or Ductal Carcinoma in Situ

One or both of your breasts may have ducts lined with cancer cells, a condition known as ductal carcinoma in situ (DCIS). The tubes known as milk ducts transport milk from your breast lobes to your nipples, enabling you to breastfeed or chest feed. Your milk ducts are where the malignancy is "in situ," or placed (contained).

Pre-invasive or non-invasive breast cancer are other terms for DCIS. This indicates that the cancer cells are still contained inside your milk duct walls. Unlike aggressive or invasive tumors, DCIS seldom metastasizes or spreads to other organs in the body.

How Common is Ductal Carcinoma in Situ (DCIS)?

DCIS, which accounts for 20% to 25% of all new cancer diagnoses each year, is a frequent form of breast cancer in women and people assigned female at birth (AFAB). DCIS can affect men and individuals who were assigned male at birth (AMAB), although it is uncommon (less than 0.1% of cancer diagnoses).

Since more people are opting to have annual mammograms to check for breast cancer, the total number of DCIS cases appears to have increased. To better detect DCIS, mammography technology has also advanced. Although it may seem unfavorable, an increase in breast cancer diagnoses is good news. More cases indicate that more people are receiving early diagnosis and treatment.

Some types of invasive breast cancer have features that affect how they develop and how they are treated:

Aggressive invasive breast cancer that tests negative for progesterone and estrogen receptors and lacks excess HER2 proteins is known as triple-negative breast cancer. Triple-negative breast cancers make up about 12% of all invasive breast cancers.

Invasive breast cancer that tests negative for TNBC is defined as follows:

- is estrogen receptor-negative, meaning it lacks receptors for the hormone estrogen.

- is progesterone receptor-negative, meaning it lacks progesterone receptors.

- does not exhibit elevated levels of the HER2 protein (sometimes referred to as HER2-negative)

Medication that targets the HER2 protein or uses hormone treatment is ineffective against triple-negative breast tumors. Ten to fifteen percent of all cases of breast cancer are triple-negative.

Triple-Negative Breast Cancer: Who Gets It?

Triple-negative breast cancer can strike anyone, but it typically strikes women who: are Black, under 40, and possess a BRCA1 mutation

Black women are twice as likely as White women to receive a triple-negative breast cancer diagnosis, according to the American Cancer Society.

Triple-positive breast cancer is characterized by an excess of HER2 proteins and positive tests for progesterone and estrogen receptors. Triple-positive breast cancers make up about 10% of all cases.

Breast cancer classified as triple-positive is one in which the HER2 protein, along with the hormone's progesterone and estrogen, drive the cancer's growth.

Triple-Positive Breast Cancer:

- estrogen receptors (positive estrogen receptors)

- progesterone receptor-positive progesterone receptors

- elevated HER2 protein levels, which function as receptors (HER2-positive)

The hormones instruct the cell to develop when they attach to their receptors. Furthermore, uncontrollably growing and dividing breast cells are caused by an excess of HER2 proteins.

For the treatment of triple-positive breast cancer, numerous medications are available. If you fall into the 10% of cases of this kind of breast cancer, your treatment approach will probably include hormone therapy, chemotherapy, and targeted therapy.

Breast Cancer Caused by Inflammation

Rapidly spreading inflammatory breast cancer (IBC) is an uncommon kind of disease. IBC rarely results in breast tissue lumps, in contrast to the majority of breast malignancies. Rather, it manifests as a rash that gives the affected breast's skin an orange peel-like feel. IBC results in dimpling, edema, redness, and pain in the afflicted breast.

IBC develops when cancerous cells obstruct lymph vessels, which are tiny, hollow tubes that let lymph fluid escape your breast. Because of the inflammation caused by the blockage, it is simple to confuse IBC for an infection.

IBC spreads quickly and needs to be treated very quickly. Chemotherapy, surgery, and radiation therapy are the usual treatments used by medical professionals for IBC.

Who is likely to have IBC, or Inflammatory Breast Cancer?

Although certain factors may increase your risk, anyone can develop inflammatory breast cancer.

Gender: Although IBC can afflict people of any gender, it is more common in women and those who were born with a female gender assignment (AFAB).

Age: Compared to those with other types of breast cancer, those with IBC typically have younger ages. The majority of women and people with AFAB who are diagnosed with inflammatory breast cancer are under 40 years old. The diagnostic age is 57 on the median.

Race: Compared to White people, Black people have a higher diagnosis rate for IBC.

Weight: Individuals who are obese or overweight have a higher diagnosis rate than those whose BMI is within normal limits.

Micro metastases

Little clusters of breast cancer cells that have spread from the breast to another part of the body, usually the lymph nodes beneath the arms, are known as micrometastases. In the lymph nodes surrounding the breast, doctors check for micrometastases because, according to research, these indicate a higher risk of breast cancer spreading and the potential need for different treatment options compared to breast cancer without micrometastases.

Metastatic breast cancer

Breast cancer that has spread to another part of the body, most frequently the bones, lungs, brain, or liver, is known as metastatic breast cancer, also known as stage IV breast cancer.

Metastasis is the term for the process by which cancer spreads. When cancer cells separate from the primary breast tumor and go to different areas of the body, this is known as metastasis. These cancer cells move via the lymphatic system, which is a network of lymph nodes and veins that get rid of viruses, germs, and cell debris.

After the initial diagnosis and course of treatment, breast cancer may recur in a different area of the body months or years later. This is referred to as a distant or metastatic recurrence. Metastatic illness affects about 30% of women with early-stage breast cancer diagnoses. males are also diagnosed with metastatic breast cancer, although the number of males with male breast cancer cases is so small that it is unclear how many of these instances go on to metastasis.

De novo metastatic breast cancer refers to breast cancer that is detected metastatically at the time of initial diagnosis. This indicates that the breast cancer has already progressed to another area of the body by the time it is initially discovered.

The cells that make up metastatic breast cancer are derived from the primary breast tumor. Therefore, breast cancer cells, not bone cancer cells, make up the metastatic tumor in the bone if breast cancer travels to the bone.

Receiving a metastatic breast cancer diagnosis can be quite stressful. Anger, fear, tension, or sadness are possible emotions. Some may have doubts about the cancer therapies they received, or they may be angry at themselves or their physicians for not being able to reverse the illness. Some people could take a matter-of-fact approach to receiving a metastatic breast cancer diagnosis. Acknowledging the diagnosis can be done in whatever way you want. You must act and feel in a way that is optimal for you and your circumstances.

Remember that there is still hope for metastatic illness. Even with stage IV breast cancer, some patients have long and fulfilling lives. For metastatic breast cancer, there are numerous treatment options available, and new medications are being evaluated daily. As they get treatment for metastatic breast cancer, an increasing number of patients are making the most of their lives.

Metastatic breast cancer cannot be cured, however, treatment can delay its progression for several years. You might be able to attempt another treatment if the first one doesn't work. The cancer may occasionally be aggressive and then enter remission. Numerous distinct therapies are frequently applied singly, in combination, or order. Your doctor may advise stopping treatment when the illness is under control and you are feeling well, depending on the circumstances.

Signs of Metastatic Breast Cancer

Depending on where the cancer has spread, the symptoms of metastatic breast cancer can vary greatly, however, several indications of the disease include:

- Persistent pain in the back, bones, or joints

- Difficulty urinating (incontinence or inability to go), which may indicate that the cancer is compressing your back nerves.

- Weakness or numbness in any part of your body

- An ongoing dry cough

- Breathing problems or shortness of breath

- Chest ache

- Diminished appetite

- Tenderness, discomfort, or bloating in the abdomen

- Persistent nausea, vomiting, or loss of weight

- Jaundice, or a yellow tint to the skin and eyelids

- Excruciating headaches

- Issues with vision (double vision, hazy vision, vision loss)

- Epilepsy

- Imbalance

- Confusion

Recurrent Breast Cancer

Invasive breast cancer that has returned months or years after therapy is known as recurrent breast cancer. Breast cancer may return locally, in adjacent lymph nodes in the armpit or collarbone, regionally, or metastatically, meaning it may spread to other parts of the body.

Signs of a Local Recurrence

Similar to those of invasive ductal carcinoma, the symptoms of a local recurrence are as follows:

- A recently discovered breast or chest wall lump

- A breast region that feels abnormally firm

The breasts swell completely or partially

o Redness or irritation of the breast area's skin
o Flattening or other alterations to the nipples
o Thickening of surgical scars; skin tugging or swelling in the vicinity of the initial breast cancer surgery site

The breast region may remain swollen and red for several months following radiation therapy and breast cancer surgery. This is typical and does not typically indicate a recurrence of breast cancer. Nevertheless, consult your physician if you observe any changes in your breasts that worry you.

You can get lumps in your restored breast due to dead fat cells or scar tissue accumulation if you underwent a mastectomy and breast reconstruction. Not only are these lumps typically not cancerous, but you should also report any breast lumps you feel to your doctor so they may be watched closely.

Breast Cancer in Men

Although it is uncommon, male breast cancer does occur. Men are diagnosed with breast cancer in less than 1% of cases. The majority of breast cancers in men are invasive ductal carcinomas.

It's a common misconception that men cannot develop breast cancer. Men can get breast cancer because they have a little bit of breast tissue, even though breast cancer is far more common in women.

The breasts of both men and women are composed of lobules (milk-producing glands), ducts (tubes that bring milk to the nipples), fatty tissue, and fibrous tissue known as stroma. Girls' bodies produce more breast tissue during puberty due to hormones. Boys' bodies produce hormones that prevent their breasts from growing, resulting in reduced breast tissue. The majority of breast cancers in men start in the milk ducts and are known as ductal carcinomas.

How Common is Breast Cancer in Men?

Breast cancer in men is an uncommon condition. Less than 1% of breast cancer cases in the US are diagnosed in men. It is anticipated that 2,710 American men will receive a breast cancer diagnosis in 2022 and that the disease will claim 530 lives. Approximately one in 1,000 men will be diagnosed with breast cancer in their lifetime, compared to one in eight women.

Regretfully, breast cancer is frequently discovered at a later stage in men. The primary cause is that, unlike women, they do not get routine screening mammography to detect breast cancer early on when treatment is more manageable. Men often aren't aware that they might develop breast cancer, so they're not aware of any changes in their breast tissue and may not know that a lump, pain, swelling, or other symptoms should be discussed with their physician.

Men should know what normal breast tissue feels and looks like, according to doctors, so they can recognize any changes. The likelihood of successfully treating breast cancer increases with early detection. Men diagnosed with breast cancer typically have similar results to women at the same age and stage of the disease.

There is less data and study explicitly devoted to male breast cancer because there are comparatively fewer cases of breast cancer in men than in women. Because of this, studies on breast cancer in women are frequently used to inform therapy decisions for male breast cancer patients.

Signs of Breast Cancer in Men

Usually, a lump in the breast that feels like a hard knot or pebble is the first indication of male breast cancer. It may take some time for men to discover a lump or other breast alteration and notify their doctor about it because most guys don't check their breasts daily and are unaware of the early warning symptoms of male breast cancer. Even though the majority of lumps are not breast cancer, you should consult a doctor as soon as you notice any unexpected changes to your breast, chest, or armpit. Early detection of breast cancer typically makes successful treatment easier.

The following are warning signs and symptoms of breast cancer in men to be aware of:

A solid lump in the breast that is frequently felt directly beneath the nipple

A bump beneath the armpit

- breast soreness
- inward-facing nipple
- clear or red discharge from the nipples

The black area surrounding the nipple called the areola, may have blisters or a rash on it.

- alterations to the skin of the breasts, like redness, dimpling, puckering, or itching
- change in the size or shape of the breast

Breast Paget Disease

An uncommon kind of breast cancer called Paget's disease appears in the skin surrounding the nipple and occasionally the areola (the darker skin that surrounds the nipple). It may be accompanied by invasive breast cancer in the same breast's milk ducts, or it may be limited to the nipple as stage 0 breast cancer (ductal carcinoma in situ). Another name for it is mammary Paget's illness.

Initially, Paget's disease of the breast may be confused for a common rash because it resembles eczema on the nipple. It could result in nipple discharge, red or elevated plaques on your skin, scaling, and itching. The majority of patients exhibiting these signs do not have Paget's disease. If you do, though, they might be the first obvious symptoms of underlying breast cancer.

Who is susceptible to breast Paget's disease?

Although rare cases have been identified in people assigned male at birth, Paget's disease of the breast primarily affects those who were assigned female at birth. Although 57 is the typical age of diagnosis, it has sometimes been detected in individuals much younger and older. Paget's disease of the breast is present in less than 4% of cases of breast cancer.

How Fast or Forcefully Does Breast Paget's Disease Progress?

That is dependent upon the presence and grade of underlying ductal cancer. "Ductal carcinoma in situ" refers to cancer that has only migrated to the milk ducts and not to the surrounding breast tissues (DCIS). This is regarded as stage 0. Radiation therapy is used after surgically removing the cancerous growth(s) and nipple.

Infiltrating or invasive ductal carcinoma is the term used to describe ductal cancer that has spread outside of the milk ducts. The cancer advances in phases. Removing the impacted breast tissue and axillary lymph nodes is still a viable treatment option in the early stages. When invasive breast cancer spreads outside of the breast, it becomes more aggressive and challenging to treat.

Breast Cancer Stages and Grades

You'll want to know the stage and grade of your breast cancer if you've been diagnosed with it. The answers will help you and your physicians make treatment decisions and learn more about what lies ahead.

There are numerous techniques for doctors to determine your breast cancer stage. Physical examinations, biopsies, X-rays, bone scans other imaging studies, and blood tests can all provide hints. To learn more, tissue samples from the breast and lymph nodes are examined under a microscope by a medical professional known as a pathologist.

Doctors use letters and numbers to determine a stage for each case of breast cancer based on these results. Although it can appear to be an odd code, it's just a means of determining the precise nature of your cancer. Consider it this way: A longer list of characters and numbers indicates a more specific diagnosis and treatment plan.

Stages of Breast Cancer

The Roman numerals I, II, III, or IV (frequently followed by A, B, or C) plus the integer zero represent the stages. Generally speaking, the cancer is more advanced the higher the number. However, it goes beyond that.

Phase 0. Early detection of the cancer has been made. It began and has remained in the milk glands or breast ducts. Learn more about stage 0 breast cancer forms and treatment choices. The term "in situ" refers to the initial location of the cancer. You're likely to hear or encounter this phrase.

Stage I: Breast cancer is referred to as invasive at this point since it has managed to escape and is now attacking healthy tissue.

When a cancer is in stage 1A, it has progressed to the fatty breast tissue. Either there may be no tumor at all, or the tumor is as big as a peanut in its shell.

Stage IB denotes the presence of a small number of cancer cells in a few lymph nodes.

Stage II: The cancer has either expanded or developed.

IIA indicates that, if there is a breast tumor at all, it is still small. It's possible that the cancer has spread to three lymph nodes or that there isn't any at all.

A stage IIB breast tumor is larger; it could resemble a lime or a walnut in size. It might not be in any lymph nodes at all.

Stage III: The cancer is thought to be advanced and more difficult to treat, but it hasn't spread to the bones or other organs.

IIIA denotes the presence of malignancy in nine or more lymph nodes extending from your collarbone to your armpit. Alternatively, it may have expanded or reached the deep breast lymph nodes. There may or may not be a big tumor in the breast in any given situation.

Even if the tumor hasn't progressed to the lymph nodes, IB indicates that it has penetrated the skin surrounding your breast or the chest wall.

IIIC denotes the presence of cancer in ten lymph nodes or more, or cancer that has spread above or below the collarbone. If there are fewer afflicted lymph nodes outside the breast but more swollen or malignant ones inside, it's likewise classified as IC.

Stage IV: The cancer has progressed to distant locations from the breast and the surrounding lymph nodes. The brain, liver, lungs, and bones are the most often affected areas. "Metastatic" refers to the fact that this stage has spread outside of the original site of the cancer.

Grades for Breast Cancer

Your doctor will want to know the grade of your cancer in addition to its stage. This allows for the measurement of the cells' appearance and growth rate of normal cells. Additionally, it will inform them of the likelihood of the disease spreading to other bodily areas. Together, the stage and grade will help them determine the most appropriate course of treatment for you and your cancer's likely prognosis.

A cancer cell's grade is determined by the degree to which it differs from normal cells. Under a microscope, they will examine three distinct cell traits and give each one a score. They use these results to determine a grade, which ranges from 1 to 3:

Grade 1 (well-differentiated): The cells are developing slowly and resemble typical breast tissue.

Grade 2 (moderately differentiated): The cells are growing a little bit quicker and have a somewhat different appearance from normal cells.

Grade 3 (poorly differentiated): The cells differ greatly from typical cells in appearance. They are likely to spread since they are expanding swiftly.

The cells in your Stage 0 ductal carcinoma in situ (DCIS) will be graded by your specialists according to their appearance. They will also check for the presence of cancer cells that are dead or dying. If so, their rate of growth is likely rapid. You have a higher grade of DCIS if there are many dead or dying cancer cells.

The TNM Breast Cancer System

Moreover, doctors classify malignancies using the letters T, N, or M. You can learn something new about your cancer from each of those letters.

Tumor, or the cancerous bulge inside the breast, is represented by the letter "T." The mass is larger or wider the higher the number following it.

"N" represents nodes, such as lymph nodes. The body is full of these tiny filters, but the area around the breast is particularly packed with them. Their purpose is to ensnare cancer cells before they spread to other bodily regions. Additionally, a number (0-III) indicates whether or not lymph nodes close to the breast have been affected by the malignancy, and if so, how many.

"M" represents metastasis. The malignancy has progressed beyond the lymph nodes and breast.

SUMMING UP

Breast cancer diagnosis often involves exams and discussions about symptoms, as well as imaging studies to examine breast tissue for abnormalities. A sample of breast tissue is taken for testing to determine if cancer is present.

A clinical breast exam involves a medical specialist checking for any unusual changes in the nipple or skin, palpating the breasts for lumps, and palpating the area under the arms and along the collarbones for bumps. Mammography is an X-ray of the breast tissue used as a screening tool, with follow-up mammography being scheduled for further detail if alarming results are found.

Breast ultrasound uses sound waves to create images of internal body components, helping the medical team determine the need for additional tests. MRI of the breast uses radio waves and a magnetic field to produce detailed images of the inside of the body.

Breast cancer comes in various forms, determined by the site of the tumor's initiation in the breast, its growth or spread, and specific characteristics that affect the tumor's behavior. Understanding the diagnosis helps select the most appropriate treatment for your particular type of breast cancer.

Invasive breast cancer, also known as invasive ductal carcinoma (IDC), is the most prevalent form, accounting for 75% of all cases. ILC, or invasive lobular carcinoma, originates in the lobules, milk-producing glands in the breast, accounting for around 10% of all invasive breast cancer cases. DCIS, or ductal carcinoma in situ, occurs when one or both breasts have ducts lined with cancer cells, allowing breastfeeding or chestfeeding.

DCIS, a frequent form of breast cancer, accounts for 20% to 25% of new cancer diagnoses each year. It can affect both women and those assigned female at birth (AFAB). The increase in DCIS cases is due to more people opting for annual mammograms and advanced mammography technology. Triple-negative breast cancer, which tests negative for progesterone and estrogen receptors and lacks excess HER2 proteins, makes up about 12% of all invasive breast cancers. It typically affects Black women, under 40, and those with a BRCA1 mutation. Triple-positive breast cancer, characterized by an excess of HER2 proteins and positive tests for progesterone and estrogen receptors, makes up about 10% of all cases. Treatment for triple-positive breast cancer includes hormone therapy, chemotherapy, and targeted therapy.

Inflammatory breast cancer (IBC) is an uncommon disease that manifests as a rash, causing dimpling, edema, redness, and pain in the affected breast. It is more common in women and those born with a female gender assignment (AFAB). IBC is more common in women and those with AFAB, with a median diagnosis of 57. Black people have a higher diagnosis rate for IBC compared to White people.

Metastatic breast cancer, also known as stage IV breast cancer, is a form of breast cancer that has spread to another part of the body, often the bones, lungs, brain, or liver. This process occurs when cancer cells separate from the primary breast tumor and move through the lymphatic system. After the initial diagnosis and treatment, breast cancer may recur in a different area, known as a distant or metastatic recurrence.

Metastatic breast cancer affects about 30% of women with early-stage diagnoses and is also diagnosed in males.

Signs of metastatic breast cancer include persistent pain in the back, bones, or joints, difficulty urinating, weakness or numbness, an ongoing dry cough, breathing problems, chest ache, diminished appetite, tenderness, nausea, vomiting, weight loss, jaundice, headaches, vision issues, epilepsy, imbalance, and confusion.

Recurrent breast cancer is invasive breast cancer that has returned months or years after therapy, either locally, regionally, or metastatically. Symptoms of a local recurrence include a recently discovered breast or chest wall lump, a breast region feeling abnormally firm, swelling, redness or irritation of the breast area's skin, flattening or alterations to the nipples, thickening of surgical scars, and skin tugging or swelling near the initial breast cancer surgery site.

In conclusion, metastatic breast cancer is a challenging condition that can be managed with various treatments and medications.

Breast cancer in men is an uncommon condition, with less than 1% of cases diagnosed in the US.

The majority of breast cancers in men are invasive ductal carcinomas, which are more common in women. Men often do not receive routine screening mammography to detect breast cancer early on, leading to a higher likelihood of being diagnosed in their lifetime.

Warning signs and symptoms of breast cancer in men include a lump in the breast, a bump beneath the armpit, breast soreness, inward-facing nipples, clear or red discharge from the nipples, alterations to the skin of the breasts, and changes in the size or shape of the breast. Paget's disease, an uncommon type of breast cancer, appears in the skin surrounding the nipple and occasionally the areola. It may be accompanied by invasive breast cancer in the same breast's milk ducts or limited to the nipple as stage 0 breast cancer (ductal carcinoma in situ).

Paget's disease progresses depending on the presence and grade of underlying ductal cancer. Stage 0 breast cancer, which has only migrated to the milk ducts and not to the surrounding breast tissues, progresses through radiation therapy after surgically removing the cancerous growth(s) and nipple. Infiltrating or invasive ductal carcinoma, which has spread outside the milk ducts, becomes more aggressive and challenging to treat.

Breast cancer stages and grades are crucial for patients to make informed treatment decisions and understand the progression of their disease. Doctors use various techniques, such as physical examinations, biopsies, X-rays, bone scans, imaging studies, and blood tests, to determine the stage of breast cancer. The stages are represented by Roman numerals I, II, III, or IV, with a higher number indicating a more specific diagnosis and treatment plan.

Stage 0 refers to early detection of breast cancer, while stage 1A indicates the cancer has progressed to fatty breast tissue. Stage IB indicates the presence of a small number of cancer cells in a few lymph nodes. Stage II indicates the cancer has either expanded or developed, while stage IIB is larger and may not be in any lymph nodes. Stage III is considered advanced and difficult to treat but hasn't spread to bones or other organs. Stage IIIA indicates the presence of cancer in nine or more lymph nodes, while Stage IV refers to the cancer spreading outside the original site.

Grades for breast cancer are determined by the degree to which cells differ from normal cells. Under a microscope, three distinct cell traits are examined and scored to determine a grade, ranging from 1 to 3. Grade 1 (well-differentiated) indicates slow growth, Grade 2 (moderately differentiated) indicates faster growth, and Grade 3 (poorly differentiated) indicates rapid growth.

The TNM Breast Cancer System classifies malignancies using letters T, N, or M, representing tumors, lymph nodes, and metastasis. Understanding these stages and grades can help doctors make more informed treatment decisions and better understand the progression of breast cancer.

CHAPTER 4: *Treatment for Breast Cancer*

Breast Cancer Treatment

Surgery to remove the malignancy is often the first step in the treatment of breast cancer. After surgery, the majority of patients with breast cancer will have additional therapies such as hormone therapy, chemotherapy, and radiation. Before surgery, some patients might get hormone therapy or chemotherapy. These drugs may lessen the cancer's size and facilitate its removal.

The specifics of your breast cancer will determine how you will be treated. Your healthcare team takes into account the cancer's stage, growth rate, and hormone sensitivity of the cancer cells. Your care team also takes into account your preferences and general health.

Treatment choices for breast cancer are numerous. Having to weigh all of your options and make difficult decisions on your treatment might be intimidating. Think about visiting a breast clinic or center to get a second opinion from a breast specialist. Speak with those who have survived breast cancer and had to make the same choice.

Breast cancer surgery

Typically, breast cancer surgery entails removing the cancer from the breast as well as a few adjacent lymph nodes. The following procedures are used to treat breast cancer:

the breast cancer is removed. A lumpectomy involves removing the cancerous breast tissue along with a portion of the surrounding healthy tissue. There is no removal of the remaining breast tissue. Wide local excision and breast-conserving surgery are other terms for this procedure. Most patients who get radiation therapy also have a lumpectomy.

A lumpectomy may be performed to remove a little tumor. Chemotherapy can sometimes be used in advance of surgery to reduce the size of the cancer and enable a lumpectomy.

eliminating every breast tissue. The surgical removal of all breast tissue is known as a mastectomy. Complete mastectomy, commonly referred to as simple mastectomy, is the most popular type of mastectomy treatment. All of the breast is removed during this treatment, including the lobules, ducts, fatty tissue, and some skin, which includes the areola and nipple.

A big cancer may be removed by a mastectomy. It may also be required if one breast has more than one cancerous region. If you are unable to have radiation therapy following surgery, or if you choose not to, you may have a mastectomy.

Some modern forms of mastectomy do not involve nipple or skin removal. For example, a mastectomy that spares some skin nevertheless leaves some skin. The areola, or surrounding skin, and the nipple remain after a mastectomy that spares the nipple. These more recent procedures can enhance the appearance of the breast following surgery, but not everyone is a good candidate for them.

Eliminating many lymph nodes. A surgery to remove a few lymph nodes for examination is called a sentinel node biopsy. Often, the surrounding lymph nodes are the initial sites where breast cancer spreads. A surgeon removes part of the lymph nodes near the cancer to check for the spread of the disease. The likelihood of discovering cancer in any of the other lymph nodes is low if none of those lymph nodes test positive for the disease. There is no need to remove any more lymph nodes.

Numerous lymph nodes being removed. Axillary lymph node dissection is a procedure used to remove a large number of armpit lymph nodes. If your imaging tests reveal that the cancer has gone to the lymph nodes, this procedure may be part of your breast cancer surgery. If a sentinel node biopsy reveals malignancy, it may also be utilized.

Taking out both breasts. Even if their other breast is cancer-free, some patients who have cancer in one breast may decide to have it removed. An operation like this is known as a contralateral prophylactic mastectomy. If you are at a high risk of developing cancer in the other breast, it may be a possibility. If you have a strong family history of cancer or if you have genetic variations that raise your risk of developing cancer, your risk may be high. The majority of patients who have one breast cancer never have another breast cancer.

Depending on the methods you select, breast cancer surgery can have complications. There is a chance of discomfort, blood, and infection with any operation. There is a chance that removing lymph nodes from the armpit will cause lymphedema or swollen arms.

After a mastectomy, you may decide to have breast reconstruction. Surgery to restore the breast's shape is known as breast reconstruction. Reconstruction with your tissue or with a breast implant are possible options. Before your breast cancer surgery, think about requesting a plastic surgeon recommendation from your medical team.

Radiation Therapy

Radiation therapy uses intense energy beams to treat cancer. Protons, X-rays, and other sources are possible sources of energy.

External beam radiation is frequently used in breast cancer treatment. You lie on a table with this kind of radiation therapy, and a machine revolves around you. The device targets certain areas of your body with radiation. It happens less frequently that radiation can enter the body. We refer to this kind of radiation as brachytherapy.

Following surgery, radiation therapy is frequently employed. Any cancer cells that may remain after surgery can be eliminated by it. The radiation reduces the cancer's chance of returning.

Radiation therapy's side effects include extreme fatigue and a sunburn-like rash in the area where the radiation is directed. Additionally, breast tissue may feel firmer or appear enlarged. More significant issues can occasionally arise. These consist of lung or cardiac damage. Rarely, the treated region may develop into a new malignancy.

Chemotherapy

Chemotherapy uses powerful medications to treat cancer. There are numerous chemotherapeutic medications available. Chemotherapy medications are frequently used in combination with treatment. Most are administered intravenously. Some come in pill form.

After surgery, chemotherapy is frequently used to treat breast cancer. It can reduce the likelihood that the cancer will return and eradicate any cancer cells that may still be present.

Chemotherapy may be administered before surgery. Chemotherapy may cause the breast cancer to shrink, making removal easier. Before surgery, chemotherapy may also help manage cancer that has progressed to the lymph nodes. Surgery to remove multiple lymph nodes may not be necessary if, following chemotherapy, the lymph nodes no longer exhibit cancerous symptoms. The medical team's decision-making about potential post-operative treatments is aided by the cancer's response to chemotherapy.

Chemotherapy can aid in the control of cancer when it spreads to other bodily parts.

Chemotherapy can help with advanced cancer symptoms including discomfort.

The adverse effects of chemotherapy vary depending on the medications you take. Hair loss, nausea, vomiting, extreme fatigue, and an elevated risk of infection are typical adverse effects. Nerve damage and early menopause are examples of uncommon adverse effects. Very rarely, blood cell cancer can be brought on by specific chemotherapy drugs.

Hormone Replacement Therapy

Medications are used in hormone therapy to block specific hormones in the body. This medication is for breast cancers that respond well to progesterone and estrogen. These malignancies are referred to the medical professionals as progesterone and estrogen receptor-positive. Hormone-sensitive cancers use their bodies' hormones as growth fuel. Reducing or eliminating the cancer cells may result from hormone-blocking.

Following surgery and other therapies, hormone therapy is frequently employed. It may lessen the chance that the cancer will return.

Hormone therapy may help control the cancer if it spreads to other bodily parts.

Hormone therapy treatments include the following:

- medications that prevent hormones from binding to cancerous cells. We refer to these medications as selective modulators of the estrogen receptor.

- drugs that prevent the body from producing estrogen beyond menopause. We refer to these medications as aromatase inhibitors.

To stop the ovaries from producing hormones, surgery or medication are used.

The adverse effects of hormone therapy vary depending on the course of treatment. Night sweats, vaginal dryness, and hot flashes are possible adverse effects. Blood clots and the possibility of bone weakening are among the more serious adverse effects.

Targeted Therapy

Utilizing medications that target particular molecules in cancer cells is known as targeted therapy. Targeted therapies can kill cancer cells by preventing these substances from functioning.

The protein HER2 is the target of the majority of targeted therapy medications for breast cancer. Certain breast cancer cells produce more HER2. This protein aids in the growth and survival of cancer cells. Drugs used in targeted therapy specifically target cells that overproduce HER2, sparing healthy cells.

There are numerous different targeted therapy medications available to treat breast cancer. To determine whether you could benefit from these medications, your cancer cells may be examined.

Before surgery, targeted treatment medications can be used to reduce the size of breast cancer and facilitate its removal. Some are used to reduce the chance of the cancer returning following surgery. Others are only applied in cases where the cancer has metastasized to other bodily regions.

Immunotherapy

Immunotherapy is a medical intervention that stimulates the immune system to eradicate cancerous cells from the body. The immune system targets bacteria and other foreign cells in the body to prevent illness. Cancer cells evade the immune system to survive. Immunotherapy aids in the immune system's ability to identify and eliminate cancerous cells.

One potential treatment option for triple-negative breast cancer is immunotherapy. Breast cancer classified as triple-negative indicates that the cancer cells lack HER2, progesterone, or estrogen receptors.

Palliative Care

When you have a terrible disease, palliative care is a unique kind of healthcare that makes you feel better. Palliative treatment can assist in reducing pain and other symptoms if you have cancer. Palliative care is given by a group of medical specialists. Physicians, nurses, and other people with specialized training may be part of the team. Enhancing your and your family's quality of life is their main objective.

Palliative care experts collaborate with you, your loved ones, and your healthcare team to promote your well-being. They offer an additional degree of assistance during your cancer treatment. Palliative care can be provided with aggressive cancer therapies including radiation therapy, chemotherapy, or surgery.

Palliative care can help cancer patients feel better and survive longer when used in conjunction with all other approved treatments.

Treatment for Breast Cancer Side Effects and How to Handle Them

The goal of breast cancer treatment is to identify and eradicate cancer cells. It differs according to the kind and stage of the disease. Breast cancer treatment is necessary and beneficial in the majority of cases, but there are potential short- and long-term negative effects from each kind of treatment. Being aware of potential side effects can help you or a loved one receiving breast cancer treatment better understand, reduce, and manage the condition.

These days, hormone therapy, targeted therapy, radiation therapy, chemotherapy, and surgery are the most often used treatments for breast cancer. The majority of therapy programs combine these choices. Side effects can differ based on the particular treatment and your personal medical history. It's important to discuss with your physician any adverse effects you may encounter, your risk factors for developing them, and ways to lessen or eliminate them.

Keep in mind that every person reacts to a cancer diagnosis, treatment, and side effects differently. What may have a significant impact on one patient may not have the same effect on another. You must stay in close communication with your healthcare team to address any adverse effects that you may experience from your therapy.

Chemotherapy, one of the most popular treatments for breast cancer, works by killing cancer cells in the body using one or more anti-cancer medications. While some side effects of chemotherapy are well-known, others are less frequent and more difficult to identify.

The most common chemo-related adverse effects, which vary depending on the kind, dosage, and duration of treatment, include:

- hair thinning

- oral sores

- Weary

- appetite decline

- vomiting and nausea

- The diarrhea

- Nail modifications

- Simple bruises

- Neuropathy causes pain and numbness in the feet and fingers

- "Chemo brain," or trouble focusing and remembering things

- decreased white blood cell numbers that increase the risk of infection

- negative effects of hormones, like:

  - Dryness in the vagina

  - Warm flashes

  - Menopause, either early or potential

  - problems with fertility

  - low level of white blood cells

  - low level of red blood cells

Handling the Side Effects of Chemotherapy

The good news is that many side effects of chemotherapy disappear when treatment is over, even though side effects can be extremely painful. There are steps you and your healthcare team can take to assist lessen some of the negative effects of chemotherapy in the interim. Always consult a medical practitioner before starting a new treatment plan.

Consume a diet that is chemo-friendly.

Chemotherapy patients frequently experience nausea, which makes it challenging to find foods that taste good and pass easily through the stomach. Focus on eating fewer meals throughout the day and choose bland foods like crackers, bread, yogurt, oatmeal, and spaghetti to help fight treatment-related nausea. There are occasions when eating or smelling peppermint can be beneficial.

Chemotherapy can also result in severe mouth sores and altered taste buds, which can make some meals taste metallic or unpleasant. Bad tastes can be eliminated by rinsing your mouth before and after eating, and the metallic aftertaste left by chemotherapy medications can be somewhat mitigated by sucking on sour or citrus-flavored sweets. To aid in the healing of certain kinds of sores, your doctor could advise you to swish a particular solution in your mouth.

It's also critical to stay hydrated to help counteract the nausea and diarrhea associated with chemotherapy by consuming lots of water, decaffeinated drinks, and juices. In the end, though, just eat what you can, when you can.

Consult your physician about anti-nausea drugs.

Chemotherapy-induced nausea is manageable with a variety of over-the-counter and prescription drugs. Most doctors will write prescriptions for nausea before your first chemotherapy treatment because they anticipate it as a side effect of the drug. However, it can be helpful to get a prescription if your doctor does not provide one before treatment.

Fill any medications your doctor provides you, and make sure you have them on hand so you can take them as directed. Ask your doctor for a different anti-nausea medicine to try if the one they gave doesn't work for you.

Combine movement or exercise with rest.

Chemotherapy frequently causes fatigue, so it's critical to give your body the rest it requires when you suffer from this side effect. However, try to get some exercise or movement in on the days when you feel like it. Stretching to ease painful muscles, going for a stroll to the mailbox or further, or even doing something useful like tidying your wardrobe can all be examples of this. Studies have indicated that engaging in physical activity can aid in pain relief, fatigue reduction, and hunger stimulation.

Get ready to lose your hair.

Hair loss is a common side effect of chemotherapy for many patients. However, the kind and amount of chemotherapy can have an impact on how severe hair loss is. Even though losing your hair can be traumatizing, planning might help lessen the shock. To try to reduce the amount of hair lost during chemotherapy, you may decide to buy a cooling cap or chop or shave your hair before it starts to come out. Recall that after chemotherapy is finished, your hair will regrow, but it can have a different texture or even color.

Side Effects of Radiation

Radiation therapy is a kind of cancer treatment that targets cancer cells with high-energy photon beams. It can be used as a stand-alone treatment or to reduce tumor size before surgery or chemotherapy.

Among the most typical adverse effects of radiation therapy for breast cancer are:

- Fatigue

- discomfort in the breasts

- swelling in the radiation-exposed area

- skin inflammation in the radiation-exposed area

As the course of treatment goes on, these adverse effects can get worse. Similar to a sunburn, the skin on and around the radiation source may feel irritated, appear red, and occasionally peel. Even after radiation, the area could still look discolored or tan.

Additionally, some persons report soreness and changes in skin sensation under their arms. Lymphedema, or swelling of the arm or upper body caused by improper lymphatic fluid drainage, is one of the more dangerous dangers.

Handling the Side Effects of Radiation

Radiation side effects, including skin irritation, can take a few weeks to manifest. You must keep your care team informed during your radiation treatments so they can provide precise recommendations on how to minimize the severity of side effects.

Apply creams and lotions.

The skin's surface is impacted by radiation's primary negative effects. As such, it's critical to maintain moisture and hydration in the area(s) that are receiving radiation. To lessen the adverse effects of radiation, try applying unscented and/or medical-grade lotions or creams to the affected area. Alternatively, contact your care team for prescription-strength creams.

Try to maintain awareness and proper sleep.

Radiation therapy can wear you out mentally and physically, much like chemotherapy does. To improve the mind-body connection during radiation treatment, make sure to take breaks from physical exertion and think about engaging in mindfulness or meditation.

Walking is a form of exercise.

Walking five times a week for thirty minutes can help reduce the side effects of weariness by over seventy percent during and after radiation treatment.

Effects of Hormone Therapy Sides

By either stopping hormones from binding to cancer cell receptors or completely stopping the synthesis of hormones, hormone therapy can be used to treat breast cancer that is sensitive to hormones like progesterone or estrogen. For individuals with hormone receptor-positive malignancies, hormone therapy is usually advised. The average duration of hormone therapy is five years or more.

Common side effects of hormone therapy include the following, though they can vary depending on the substance or kind used:

- Warm flashes

- Dryness in the vagina

- Sweats at night

- Joint and muscle soreness

- The osteoporosis

- Gaining weight

- Headaches

- emesis

- Weary

- Changes in mood

- Low desire

Hormone therapy can also have an impact on a woman's menstrual cycle, occasionally resulting in irregular menstruation or, in premenopausal women, menopause.

Handling the Side Effects of Hormone Therapy

While a woman may have certain short-term adverse effects from hormone therapy, many other side problems could last for the remainder of her life. It's critical to collaborate with your doctor to try and control any short- or long-term negative effects you may have. Here are some more strategies to deal with side effects.

Consume a wholesome, balanced diet.

The fuel you need to recover and maintain your health comes from a balanced diet. Additionally, it can lessen the negative effects of cancer treatment.

Continue to move and exercise to stay active.

Osteoporosis, weight gain, and joint and muscular pain are typical long-term side effects of hormone therapy. Try to include exercise or movement in your everyday routine to counter this. Research indicates that engaging in 150 minutes of physical activity each week, or roughly 20 minutes daily, may aid in mitigating the intensity of these typical adverse effects.

Apply moisturizers or lubricants to the vagina.

When vaginal dryness becomes uncomfortable or painful during sexual activity, consider using water-soluble vaginal lubricants before engaging in sexual activity. Get in touch with your gynecologist if discomfort or dryness persists. Regular usage of vaginal moisturizers can help to keep the vaginal wall healthy. Certain physicians may even recommend taking a very little amount of estrogen twice a week in the form of vaginal tablets called Estrodiol. It can repair the vaginal wall and has extremely little blood absorption.

Give up smoking and consume less alcohol.

Drinking alcohol and smoking both have detrimental consequences on health, particularly for those who are coping with or have survived breast cancer. Reducing drinking and smoking might help you feel better overall, which can lessen the severity of side effects after treatment. Moreover, it lowers the chance of a recurrence of breast cancer.

Consult your physician about taking natural supplements.

Numerous natural supplements can help lessen the negative effects of hormone therapy, including probiotics, calcium, magnesium, and vitamin D. Before incorporating additional vitamins or supplements into your treatment regimen, discuss any possible drug interactions with your doctor.

Side Effects of Targeted Therapy

Targeted therapy is a more recent method for treating breast cancer. It involves the use of medications that, by selectively targeting certain proteins in breast cancer cells, can stop the growth of these cells without endangering healthy cells. Chemotherapy is frequently combined with it; certain adverse effects are similar to chemotherapy, while others are distinct. Among them are:

- vomiting and nausea

- Weary

- The diarrhea

- oral sores

- Dry skin and/or rashes

- Neuropathy causes pain and numbness in the feet and fingers

- alterations in the heart

Throughout treatment, your doctor will also keep an eye out for any indications of liver, heart, lung, or clotting problems.

Handling the Side Effects of Targeted Therapy

Similar to chemotherapy, the kind of therapy being received and its duration affects the degree and duration of side effects associated with targeted therapy. It's crucial to discuss the potential adverse effects of targeted therapy with your physician or care team, as well as strategies for handling them as they arise during your course of treatment.

Heart tests are performed on women receiving biologic-targeted therapy for HER2+ breast cancer regularly to assist make sure no cardiac side effects are occurring. Up to ten years after the last therapy, patients may experience cardiac side effects from this class of medications.

Adverse Effects of Surgery

Surgery, which includes lumpectomy, mastectomy, breast reconstruction, and lymph node excision, is still the most prevalent treatment for breast cancer. As with any surgery, stiffness, edema, pain, and discomfort are possible side effects.

Additional possible adverse consequences of surgery for breast cancer include:

- nerve discomfort

- Weary

- Modification of feeling in the vicinity of the surgical site

- Alterations to the skin and bruises

- emesis

- At the surgical site, scar tissue

- edema lymphatic

You should call your doctor right away if you have any of the following symptoms soon after surgery: warm-to-the-touch wound, increased temperature, or fluid discharge from the surgical site.

Handling Post-Surgery Side Effects

During the post-operative phase, you must adhere to all directions given by your surgeon and care staff. This includes attending surgical follow-up appointments, taking all prescription medications as instructed, and taking proper care of the wound site.

Physical therapy and stretching

After receiving the all-clear and being discharged from your surgeon's care, consult your doctor or the care team again for any stretches or exercises that are necessary to improve your range of motion and prevent the surgical site from stiffening up, or "cording." To do this, your doctor might advise you to include a physical therapist on your care team. Pain relief, reduced fatigue, and increased appetite are all possible with physical therapy. You may also include massage and acupuncture in your toolbox for post-operative recovery.

Your care team or a physical therapist can also assist you in managing the symptoms of lymphedema by providing expert massages or fitting you with a compression sleeve specifically designed for the affected area.

Women who have a mastectomy without reconstructive surgery may feel pain or have phantom limbs. The breast is regarded by the brain similarly to an arm or leg. People who have had limbs amputated may remark that they "still feel" the amputated limb or that it hurts or feels hot. After a mastectomy, the same symptoms may appear. Scratching under the arms has been shown to help reduce phantom limb sensation, which is experienced by women who have had mastectomies yet still have nipple irritation. Phantom breast pain or sensation can also be lessened or mitigated by wearing a breast prosthesis.

SUMMING UP

Breast cancer treatment typically begins with surgery to remove the malignancy. Following surgery, patients often receive additional therapies such as hormone therapy, chemotherapy, and radiation. The specifics of the cancer determine the treatment, which may include hormone therapy or chemotherapy to reduce the cancer's size.

There are numerous treatment options for breast cancer, including lumpectomy, mastectomy, sentinel node biopsy, axillary lymph node dissection, and contralateral prophylactic mastectomy. A lumpectomy involves removing the cancerous breast tissue along with a portion of the surrounding healthy tissue. A mastectomy can be performed for large or multiple cancerous regions, and some modern forms may not involve skin removal. Sentinel node biopsy is a surgical procedure to remove part of the lymph nodes near the cancer to check for disease spread. Axillary lymph node dissection is a procedure used to remove a large number of armpit lymph nodes.

After a mastectomy, patients may decide to have breast reconstruction to restore the breast's shape. Reconstruction with tissue or a breast implant is possible, and it is important to request a plastic surgeon recommendation from your medical team.

Radiation therapy uses intense energy beams to treat cancer, such as protons, X-rays, and other sources. External beam radiation, also known as brachytherapy, is commonly used in breast cancer treatment. Post-surgery, radiation therapy is often used to eliminate any remaining cancer cells and reduce the cancer's chance of returning. Side effects of radiation therapy include fatigue, sunburn-like rash, firmer breast tissue, lung or cardiac damage, and rare cases of new malignancy.

Chemotherapy is a powerful treatment for breast cancer, using powerful medications to reduce the likelihood of the cancer returning and eradicate any remaining cells. It can be administered before surgery or before surgery to shrink the breast cancer and manage cancer that has progressed to the lymph nodes. Chemotherapy can help control cancer when it spreads to other body parts and manage advanced symptoms.

Hormone therapy is used to block specific hormones in the body, targeting progesterone and estrogen receptor-positive breast cancers. It may also help control the cancer if it spreads to other bodily parts. Adverse effects of hormone therapy include hair loss, nausea, vomiting, extreme fatigue, an elevated risk of infection, nerve damage, early menopause, and blood cell cancer.

Targeted therapy targets specific molecules in cancer cells, specifically targeting the protein HER2, which aids in the growth and survival of cancer cells. There are numerous different targeted therapy medications available, and some are used before surgery to reduce the size of breast cancer and facilitate its removal.

Immunotherapy is a medical intervention that stimulates the immune system to eradicate cancerous cells from the body. It can be provided with aggressive cancer therapies like radiation therapy, chemotherapy, or surgery. Palliative care is a unique form of healthcare that helps cancer patients feel better and survive longer when used in conjunction with all other approved treatments.

Being aware of potential side effects can help you understand, reduce, and manage the condition. Most common treatments for breast cancer include hormone therapy, targeted therapy, radiation therapy, chemotherapy, and surgery. It is important to discuss any adverse effects with your physician and stay in close communication with your healthcare team.

Chemotherapy is a popular treatment for breast cancer that uses anti-cancer medications to kill cancer cells. Common side effects include hair thinning, oral sores, weariness, appetite decline, vomiting and nausea, diarrhea, nail changes, simple bruises, neuropathy, decreased white blood cell numbers, negative effects of hormones, dryness in the vagina, warm flashes, menopause, fertility problems, and low levels of white and red blood cells.

To manage these side effects, consult a medical practitioner before starting a new treatment plan. Consume a diet that is chemo-friendly, stay hydrated, and consult your physician about anti-nausea drugs. Combining movement or exercise with rest can help reduce fatigue and pain.

Hair loss is a common side effect of chemotherapy, but planning can help lessen the shock. Consider buying a cooling cap, cutting, or shaving your hair before it starts to grow.

Radiation therapy targets cancer cells with high-energy photon beams and can cause fatigue, discomfort, swelling, and skin inflammation. Keep your care team informed during radiation treatments to provide precise recommendations on how to minimize the severity of side effects. Apply creams and lotions to maintain moisture and hydration in the affected area.

Maintain awareness and proper sleep to improve the mind-body connection during radiation treatment. Engage in mindfulness or meditation to improve the mind-body connection. Walking five times a week for thirty minutes can help reduce weariness side effects by over seventy percent during and after radiation treatment.

Hormone therapy is a treatment for breast cancer that targets hormone receptors, such as progesterone or estrogen. It typically lasts five years or more and can cause common side effects such as warm flashes, vagina dryness, night sweats, joint and muscle soreness, osteoporosis, weight gain, headaches, emesis, wearyness, mood changes, and low desire. These side effects can also impact a woman's menstrual cycle.

To manage these side effects, it is essential to consume a balanced diet, stay active, apply moisturizers or lubricants to the vagina, give up smoking and consume less alcohol, and consult your physician about taking natural supplements. Targeted therapy, a more recent method, uses medications to selectively target certain proteins in breast cancer cells without endangering healthy cells. It can cause symptoms similar to chemotherapy but with distinct side effects.

Surgery, including lumpectomy, mastectomy, breast reconstruction, and lymph node excision, is still the most common treatment for breast cancer. Side effects include stiffness, edema, pain, and discomfort, nerve discomfort, alterations to the skin and bruises, emesis, scar tissue, and edema lymphatic.

Post-surgery side effects include adhering to surgeon and care staff's directions, taking prescribed medications, and proper wound site care. Physical therapy and stretching can help improve range of motion and prevent stiffening up of the surgical site. Physical therapists may be recommended for pain relief, reduced fatigue, and increased appetite.

Women who have had a mastectomy without reconstructive surgery may experience pain or have phantom limbs, which can be alleviated by wearing a breast prosthesis. It is crucial to consult with a doctor and care team to manage these side effects effectively.